Program Collaboration and Service Integration:

Enhancing the Prevention and Control of HIV/AIDS,
Viral Hepatitis, Sexually Transmitted Diseases, and
Tuberculosis in the United States

An NCHHSTP White Paper, 2009

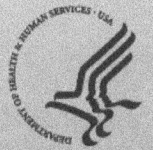

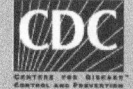

U.S. DEPARTMENT OF HEALTH AND HUMAN SERVICES
CENTERS FOR DISEASE CONTROL AND PREVENTION

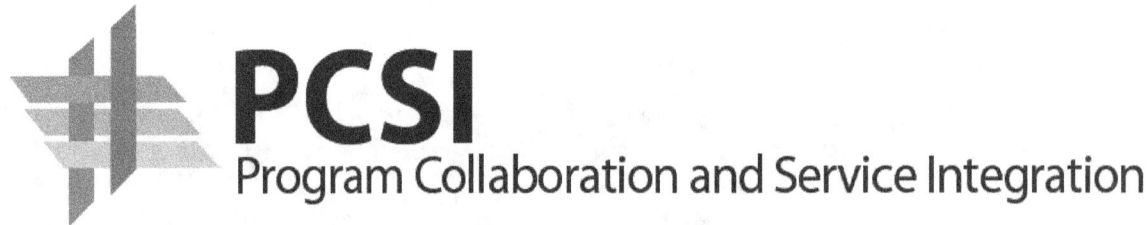

PCSI
Program Collaboration and Service Integration

Suggested Citation: Centers for Disease Control and Prevention. Program Collaboration and
Service Integration: Enhancing the Prevention and Control of HIV/AIDS, Viral Hepatitis,
Sexually Transmitted Diseases, and Tuberculosis in the United States.
Atlanta (GA): U.S. Department of Health and Human Services, Centers for Disease Control and Prevention; 2009.

TABLE OF CONTENTS

EXECUTIVE SUMMARY

Single, categorical services provided to persons with multiple related risks miss significant opportunities to diagnose, treat, and prevent disease.[1] This is exacerbated in communities that are considered "hard to reach." Small changes in the way prevention services are delivered can make a dramatic difference by reaching a larger population with more services. It can also improve efficiency, cost-effectiveness and health outcomes.

CDC's National Center for HIV/AIDS, Viral Hepatitis, STD, and TB Prevention's (NCHHSTP) program collaboration and service integration (PCSI) strategic priority is working to strengthen collaborative work across disease areas and integrate services that are provided by related programs, especially prevention activities related to HIV/AIDS, viral hepatitis, other sexually transmitted diseases (STDs), and tuberculosis (TB) at the client level. PCSI is a mechanism for organizing and blending interrelated health issues, activities, and prevention strategies to facilitate a comprehensive delivery of services. There are five principles that form the decision making framework for PCSI: appropriateness, effectiveness, flexibility, accountability, and acceptability. By following these five principles for PCSI, programs can deliver more comprehensive integrated services to identify and treat disease more effectively to improve the health outcomes of the persons they serve.

PCSI combines two approaches for improving public health outcomes: program collaboration and service integration. Program Collaboration involves a mutually beneficial and well-defined relationship between two or more programs, organizations, or organizational units to achieve common goals. It involves many aspects of comprehensive program management at state and local levels; the 10 essential public health functions, developed by the Core Public Health Functions Steering Committee in 1994, provide a useful framework for categorizing collaboration strategies among programs (Table 1).

Service Integration provides persons with seamless comprehensive services from multiple programs without repeated registration procedures, waiting periods, or other administrative barriers. NCHHSTP describes three levels of service integration at the client–provider interface: nonintegrated services, core integrated services, and expanded integrated services (Table 2). "Core" integrated services are combinations of services for which CDC has published guidance or recommendations, and "expanded" integrated services are best and promising evidence-based practice for which CDC has not yet published specific guidance.

NCHHSTP is committed to supporting PCSI efforts initiated by staff, grantees, and partners. The use of PCSI as a structural intervention by CDC's national, state and local partners will help achieve multiple related health goals to appropriate populations whenever they interact with the health system.

Small changes in the way services are delivered have the potential to maximize prevention opportunities.

The five principles of effective PCSI

- *appropriateness*
- *effectiveness*
- *flexibility*
- *accountability*
- *acceptability*

Partners should utilize PCSI as a structural intervention to provide comprehensive, evidence-based care and prevention services.

This white paper outlines NCHHSTP's strategic vision for program collaboration and service integration, building on and refining concepts outlined in a 2007 green paper. This earlier paper presented a framework for service integration and introduced the concept of PCSI "levels of integration" as a way to conceptualize, implement, and deliver holistic, evidence-based prevention services and risk reduction messages to appropriate populations in clinical settings. As a document used to communicate NCHHSTP policy, this white paper

- defines and articulates a framework for conceptualizing PCSI
- identifies how NCHHSTP will work with internal and external stakeholders to accomplish relevant goals
- outlines key measures to monitor and evaluate progress
- describes how NCHHSTP will work with partners at national, state, and local levels to advance PCSI

The primary intended audience for this document is state and local health departments, community based organizations and other domestic partners that are directly or indirectly funded by NCHHSTP. The document describes NCHHSTP policy, and thus has implications for other CDC units, federal agencies, publicly funded agencies and organizations, hospitals, community health centers, professional organizations, and private health-care providers whose management, program objectives, populations, sites, or services intersect significantly with those of NCHHSTP.

INTRODUCTION

Background

For years, many national organizations and CDC grantees have called for better integration of services that are provided by related programs, especially of prevention activities related to HIV/AIDS, other sexually transmitted diseases (STDs), viral hepatitis, and tuberculosis (TB).[2-6] Public health leaders, care providers, and prevention partners continually strive to increase their ability to respond to changing disease epidemiology, eliminate missed opportunities, and meet the needs of communities and populations at risk for multiple infections. As early as 1998, the Advisory Committee for HIV and STD Prevention recommended that CDC include early STD detection and treatment as an explicit component of comprehensive HIV prevention programs at national, state and local levels.[7]

Several factors have accelerated the momentum toward collaboration and integration of prevention services related to the epidemics of HIV, other STDs, viral hepatitis, and TB in the United States. One factor is our greater understanding of the extent to which these diseases are synergistically interacting epidemics or syndemics.[8] The risk of acquiring any of these diseases is associated with similar behaviors and environmental conditions, and they have reciprocal or interdependent effects. For example,

- HIV, viral hepatitis and STDs share common risks and modes of transmission;
- STDs increase the risk for HIV infection;
- HIV is the greatest risk factor for progression to TB disease;
- TB is an AIDS-defining opportunistic condition; and
- Clinical course and outcomes are influenced by concurrent disease (HIV/TB can be deadly, and TB accelerates HIV disease progression).

As a result, certain populations are at elevated risk for multiple diseases.

Common risks suggest the need for common solutions and enhanced collaboration among related prevention programs. Because these disease conditions share many social, environmental, behavioral, and biological determinants and are often managed by the same or similar organizations, public health efforts to prevent their occurrence require a syndemic orientation. This provides a way of thinking about public health work that focuses on connections among health-related problems, considers those connections when developing health policies and aligns public health activities with other avenues of social change to foster conditions in which all people can be healthy.[8]

The usual public health approach to disease prevention often begins by defining the disease in question; a syndemic-oriented approach first defines the population in question, identifies the conditions that create and sustain health in that population, examines why those conditions might differ among groups and determines how those conditions might be addressed in a comprehensive manner.[8]

Public health leaders, care providers, and prevention partners are continually striving to better address the needs of communities and populations at risk for multiple infections.

Common risks suggest the need for common solutions and enhanced collaboration among related prevention programs.

A key benefit of service integration is that it encourages service providers to offer various interrelated services to persons whenever they access services.

The focus on PCSI is the desire of CDC and its partners to ensure that individuals receive the best preventive service and treatment possible whenever they interact with providers of health services.[2-6,9-11] A key benefit of service integration is that it encourages service providers to offer various interrelated services to persons whenever they access services. In many ways, local-level service providers have led the way in recognizing the need for improved collaboration among prevention programs and in integrating appropriate services.[2-6,10-13]

Understanding the local epidemiology, as well as understanding risks and the service needs of the communities served are essential components of developing appropriate, comprehensive services and thereby enhancing quality, public health impact and cost-effectiveness.

New CDC recommendations and advances in diagnostic technology have greatly decreased barriers and facilitated the provision of integrated services. The advent of new recommendations for partner services and routine HIV testing in clinical settings, as well as noninvasive urine-based testing for chlamydia and gonorrhea, for example, have made service integration more feasible than ever in traditional settings such as STD, family planning, and TB clinics. Service integration is also feasible in other settings such as community health centers, correctional and juvenile detention facilities, prenatal clinics, drug treatment centers, and hospital emergency departments.[14-18]

A final reason for the growing PCSI momentum is that limited and dwindling federal resources for core program activities make integration of prevention activities and efficiency in service delivery critically important. NCHHSTP and its partners believe that the public health benefits of PCSI can be increased by eliminating duplicative services, streamlining services, developing a workforce trained in the delivery of integrated services, and aligning systems to achieve maximum public health benefit.[10-12,19]

Understanding the local epidemiology, as well as understanding risks and the service needs of the communities served are essential components of developing appropriate, comprehensive services.

PCSI Green Paper

In 2007, NCHHSTP issued a green paper (a discussion document intended to stimulate debate and launch a process of consultation) on PCSI.[20] The paper described the rationale for PCSI, a framework for service integration, and NCHHSTP commitment to work with partners to foster PCSI. The green paper introduced the concept of PCSI "levels of integration" as a way to conceptualize, implement, and deliver holistic, evidence-based prevention services and risk reduction messages to appropriate populations in clinical settings. This white paper builds upon and refines the concepts presented in the green paper.

PCSI External Consultation

In late August 2007, NCHHSTP convened an external consultation to engage key internal and external stakeholders in developing and refining the PCSI objectives and priorities presented in the green paper.[19] Meeting participants included NCHHSTP leadership and staff and representatives from 40 state and local HIV, viral hepatitis, STD, and TB programs; other federal agencies; national organizations; and community-based organizations funded by NCHHSTP. The purpose of the meeting was to engage key stakeholders in developing and refining NCHHSTP's PCSI vision and PCSI objectives and to obtain consensus on priorities for NCHHSTP's PCSI activities over the next 5 years. Participants were asked to comment on and confirm the framing of PCSI as outlined in the green paper, identify what NCHHSTP can do to assist local PCSI efforts, and identify what they can do to improve their own PCSI efforts.

Participants were asked to work in small groups to identify the top three priorities for each of the following: (1) opportunities for PCSI implementation, (2) policy improvements needed in support of PCSI, (3) performance measures with which to assess levels of service integration, and (4) workforce development and training needs in support of PCSI. A full copy of the PCSI external consultation report is available at http://www.cdc.gov/nchhstp/programintegration/. A summary of the key findings recommendations from the meeting is in Appendix 1.

This white paper builds upon and refines the concepts presented in the green paper.

PROGRAM COLLABORATION AND SERVICE INTEGRATION

Definition: Program collaboration and service integration is a mechanism for organizing and blending interrelated health issues, activities, and prevention strategies to facilitate comprehensive delivery of services.

Vision: CDC is committed to improving people's lives by maximizing the health impact of public health services, reducing disease prevalence and promoting health equity. NCHHSTP will look broadly across program areas to implement naturally synergistic ways to collaborate and use resources wisely, using epidemiologic data to identify opportunities to intervene in the transmission of multiple infections in a coordinated way. NCHHSTP will build on existing best practices and find new ways to foster collaborative work, expand programmatic flexibility, and facilitate the appropriate integration of service delivery at the local level.

Rationale: The rationale for PCSI is to maximize the health benefits that persons receive from prevention services by increasing service efficiency by combining, streamlining, and enhancing prevention services; maximizing opportunities to screen, test, treat, or vaccinate those in need of these services; improving the health of populations negatively affected by multiple diseases; and enabling service providers to adapt to and keep pace with changes in disease epidemiology and new technologies.

PCSI should be considered a structural intervention and a crucial step toward the achievement of multiple related health goals. It provides a framework for addressing connected health-related problems and for consideration of those connections during the development of health policies, prevention programs, risk reduction messages, interventions, and research.

A major prerequisite for effective PCSI is having participating programs define and agree on common purposes and strategies. In NCHHSTP, all programs share the goal of promoting health equity related to HIV, viral hepatitis, STD, and TB infections. Other common goals across NCHHSTP programs include the following:

- Preventing infection and disease among persons at risk;
- Interrupting disease transmission through prompt diagnosis and adequate treatment;
- Ensuring access to high-quality, culturally appropriate services and key messages for marginalized, underinsured and uninsured at-risk populations;
- Monitoring infections in the population (e.g., case surveillance);
- Ensuring that healthcare systems maintain patient confidentiality; and
- Managing and reducing stigma associated with these infections and the consequences of such stigma to those accessing services and to those providing them.

PCSI is a mechanism for organizing and blending interrelated health issues, activities, and prevention strategies to facilitate comprehensive delivery of services.

CDC is committed to improving people's lives by maximizing the health impact of public health services on reducing disease prevalence and promoting health equity.

PCSI is made easier
by the use of
similar prevention
tools across programs

By integrating
related services
provided to
underserved
populations, PCSI
may also be a key
strategy for
increasing health
equity.

PCSI is made easier by the use of similar prevention tools across programs. NCHHSTP programs all employ the methods of patient counseling, partner identification and partner services, disease treatment, referrals to other services and activities designed to change behaviors, such as social marketing campaigns. The use of PCSI in the delivery of clinical services by multiple programs is also enhanced if programs serve common target populations and engage in similar activities.

Similarly, the use of PCSI in correctional institutions is facilitated by the homogeneity of the incarcerated population, access to inmates, and having a common service provider for inmates. The importance of adopting PCSI in correctional institutions is illustrated by the impact of disease transmission both within the correctional setting and in the community when inmates with undiagnosed infection(s) are released.

The goal of improved sexual health, shared by most NCHHSTP programs, also contributes to the center's use of PCSI to provide comprehensive holistic services (including risk reduction messages, mental health, substance abuse prevention and treatment, and reproductive health services) as part of a package of evidence-based preventive care to those at greatest risk for disease.

Five Principles of Effective Program Collaboration and Service Integration

Appropriateness

The integration of prevention services must make epidemiologic and programmatic sense and should be contextually appropriate. Not everyone is at risk for all diseases, and not all settings have a high prevalence of all conditions. For example, CDC currently recommends that all patients initiating treatment for TB should be screened routinely for HIV infection.[21] However, integrating comprehensive STD services with TB treatment may be neither desirable nor feasible for all TB patients. In complex outbreaks, such as that involving HIV-infected TB patients with unnamed, potentially HIV-positive contacts, collaboration among STD, HIV/AIDS, and TB programs, including activities related to contact investigation and cross-matching of databases, would clearly be appropriate.

Effectiveness

Prevention resources are far too limited to be wasted on ineffective or unproven interventions or settings. Routine HIV testing and provision of hepatitis A and B vaccinations are examples of interventions that have proved to be effective and should be expanded. Additionally, offering of vaccination services may be used as an incentive to increase uptake of HIV testing or behavioral interventions. Programs should monitor effectiveness and yield of new diagnoses resulting from service integration. As disease conditions evolve, changes are continually needed in the combination or structure of services to optimize yield. Such integration of services and monitoring would improve effectiveness and enable local providers to leverage the investments they have already made through efficiencies in service delivery.

Flexibility

Health organizations need the ability to respond to changes in disease epidemiology, demographic changes, advances in technology, and policy/political imperatives. Effective PCSI initiatives would help health organizations to consistently examine and revise how integration of services could best meet their populations' needs. If an integrated service is no longer effective in maximizing opportunities for prevention, flexibility is needed to identify more effective settings or services to accomplish this requirement. Operational changes can be made faster, more cheaply, and with a higher degree of quality when processes and services can be adapted by making minor modifications to existing programs.

Accountability

Prevention partners need the ability to monitor key aspects of their prevention services and gain insight into how they can optimize operations to maximize opportunities for prevention. NCHHSTP views PCSI as a means by which to improve the quality of prevention services. By tracking appropriate indicators that reflect operational performance and comparing them against previously defined key performance standards, NCHHSTP's partners can create a continuous feedback loop that facilitates iterative process improvement.

Acceptability

To be effective, PCSI must be accepted by program staff members and service providers, as well as by the persons they serve. The objective of PCSI is not to provide additional disjointed services that needlessly burden the provider. Rather, PCSI should empower the provider to provide all the services that are needed, thereby increasing the health and satisfaction of service recipients. For example, there is evidence that offering hepatitis vaccination may increase acceptance of STD and HIV testing and other prevention services.[22, 23]

PROGRAM COLLABORATION

Definition: Program collaboration is a mutually beneficial and well-defined relationship entered into by two or more programs, organizations, or organizational units to achieve common goals. The collaborative relationship usually includes a commitment to mutual relationships and goals, a jointly developed structure, shared responsibility, mutual authority and accountability for success, and sharing of resources and rewards.[24]

Rationale: Collaborations can broaden the mission of member organizations and help them develop more comprehensive strategies; help develop wider public support for issues and increase the influence that individuals, communities, and institutions have over community policies and practices; minimize duplication of services and increase the efficiency with which financial and human resources are used; increase participation from diverse sectors and constituencies; make the most of new resources in a changing environment; increase program accountability and planning and evaluation capacity; and increase the ability of local organizations and institutions to respond better to the needs and aspirations of their constituents.[25]

While program collaboration is not always expected to lead directly to integrated services at the client level, it can be used to do so. Program collaboration may also be used to strengthen programs by increasing access to different types of information or expertise. It can reduce program costs through joint funding of activities important to multiple programs, and to monitor the success of these activities. For example, analysis of surveillance and case-management data across programs can help staff from all participating programs keep abreast of the changing epidemiology of diseases, disease risks, and population subgroups most at risk for diseases, thereby better targeting interventions and prevention services.

Sharing of data can also help identify emerging trends that require adjustments in program activities. For example, data sharing can help identify an increase in rates of other STDs among HIV-positive persons who find partners on the Internet, a finding that would indicate a need for increased STD prevention services for that population.

Program collaboration is a mutually beneficial and well-defined relationship entered into by two or more programs, organizations, or organizational units to achieve common goals.

A Framework for Collaboration

Opportunities for greater collaboration that could enhance integrated approaches to service delivery involve many aspects of comprehensive program management at state and local levels. The 10 essential public health functions,[26] developed by the U.S. Public Health Service Core Public Health Functions Steering Committee in 1994, provide a useful framework for categorizing strategies that could be enhanced by collaboration among programs. Table 1 lists the 10 essential public health functions and provides examples of collaboration strategies and evaluation process measures.

Program collaboration facilitates joint planning and sharing or coordination of resources to the extent necessary to provide more holistic prevention services and risk reduction messages to individuals. That a single public health worker may be working with an individual or family with multiple conditions (e.g., TB, HIV, and hepatitis C) underscores the need for cross-training of personnel as well as for coordinated funding of these positions.

Program collaboration can be used to plan for, and in some cases provide, integrated services. One example of collaborative planning for service integration is holding discussions with laboratory managers so that efficient diagnostic solutions can be provided as a foundation for surveillance and client services. Another example is the collaboration of several agencies in the development of a "one-stop shop," where service providers from multiple agencies (e.g., disease prevention, family planning, welfare/housing assistance, and mental health) are co-located and share costs for administrative personnel and other infrastructure common to all agencies. The U.S. Government Accountability Office (GAO) has identified several activities necessary for successful service integration and collaboration.[27] These include

- Gaining support from key officials and stakeholders and encouraging participation and cooperation;

- Developing a "common vision" to increase agreement on goals and strategies; and

- Identifying common needs of individuals to collaboratively reduce duplication of efforts.

10 Essential Public Health Functions

- *Monitor*
- *Diagnose and investigate*
- *Inform and educate*
- *Mobilize*
- *Develop policies and plans*
- *Enforce*
- *Link*
- *Assure*
- *Evaluate*
- *Research*

Table 1. Essential Public Health Functions and Potential Collaboration Strategies Among Programs.

Program Function	Examples of Potential Collaboration Strategies	Examples of Process Measures
1. Monitor community members' health status to identify and solve community health problems.	• Develop shared vision and mutually beneficial agreements that lead to enhanced surveillance and evaluation capacity (e.g., reduce redundant systems, track comorbidity) or capability (e.g., provide cross-training for data managers). • Develop operating procedures and agreements that ensure each program has access to relevant data sets (e.g., surveillance, case management) needed for public health action. • Develop common reporting and data-collection instruments. • Conduct two-way data registry matching and analyses looking across data sets for relevant trends. • Link data sets to allow programs and researchers to assess the relationship between common risk factors and multiple specific outcomes. • Develop and disseminate cross-program reports and briefs.	• Procedures are in place for data sharing. • Programs are using shared data. • Data sets are established and analyses have been prioritized.
2. Diagnose and investigate health problems and health hazards in the community.	• Identify populations and settings that are a high priority for multiple programs, and develop a joint approach to providing outreach, testing, and risk-reduction services. (See Table 2 for PCSI levels of service integration.)	• A working group has been established. • Necessary data and analyses have been identified and requested.
3. Inform, educate, and empower people about health issues.	• Develop communication channels and consider novel communication strategies like health information technology that improve information flow between and within programs. • Identify partners working with multiple infectious disease programs, and coordinate common activities. • Develop and test integrated prevention messages for diseases with common risk factors. • Develop messages that address cross-cutting infectious disease priorities. • Develop web-based information and provide links to multiple relevant program services.	• Partners have been identified and contacted, and a system has been established. • Research or evaluation design to test messages has been developed. • Messages have been developed. • Web-based information has been developed or enhanced.
4. Mobilize community partnerships and action to identify and solve health problems.	• Develop local or regional partnerships and coalitions that have broad representation from areas affected by multiple infectious diseases with common routes of transmission. • Ensure targeted communities are represented in planning, implementation, and evaluation of activities across programs. • Work with community partners and contacts jointly across programs.	• A coalition has been established, and a working charter has been agreed upon. • Communities/affected populations from all programs are represented in the coalition.
5. Develop policies and plans that support individual and community health efforts.	• Develop and advocate for the integration of policies related to multiple commonly acquired infectious diseases and risk factors. • Develop cross-program individual, group, and community-level interventions. • Revise policies and regulations to facilitate a collaborative response to interrelated public health issues and service integration.	• A system is in place to regularly review and address policies to facilitate improved PCSI. • Cross-program interventions are being developed. • Newly developed policies and regulations remove barriers to program effectiveness.
6. Enforce laws and regulations that protect people's health and ensure their safety.	• Review the development and implementation of laws and regulations that support effective structural interventions to prevent HIV/AIDS, viral hepatitis, STD, and TB infections. • Assess policies and update those that may be barriers to program effectiveness.	• A system is in place to regularly review and address structural facilitators and barriers. • Outdated policies and legal barriers are removed.
7. Link people to needed personal health services.	• Identify opportunities for integrated prevention programs, risk reduction messages and testing where individuals, groups, or networks would benefit from counseling and testing for two or more diseases (e.g., HIV/AIDS, viral hepatitis, STD, and TB) in a clinical, behavioral intervention or outreach setting. • Collaborate with internal and external partners involved in all aspects of partner services; ensure that partner services are offered and accessible throughout the prevention and care continuum.	• Enhanced partner services are offered. • Testing is offered for multiple diseases.
8. Ensure the competency of the public and personal healthcare workforce.	• Cross-train front-line staff to identify risk factors or other diseases, or make referrals for further evaluation when appropriate. • Cross-train staff to conduct testing, screening, and partner services. • Develop internal cross-program communication mechanisms to keep all staff up-to-date on all programs.	• Training is available and being used, or training is being developed. • Cross-program communication mechanisms have been established, and their usefulness is being assessed.
9. Evaluate the effectiveness, accessibility, and quality of personal and population-based health services.	• Develop mechanisms to track the outcomes of combined interventions. • Determine the population-level impact of PCSI on HIV/AIDS, viral hepatitis, STD, and TB prevention.	• A tracking mechanism has been developed. • Funding has been identified for research on the population-level impact of PCSI. • Client/patient satisfaction is being evaluated.
10. Conduct research to identify innovative solutions to health problems.	• Identify and support research to devise effective PCSI models.	• Research collaboration has been established.

SERVICE INTEGRATION

Definition: Service integration is a distinct method of service delivery that provides persons with seamless services from multiple programs or areas within programs without repeated registration procedures, waiting period or other administrative barriers. It differs from system coordination, in which services from multiple agencies are provided but persons may have to visit different locations and register separately for each agency's programs to obtain these services.[28]

Rationale: The objective of service integration is to provide key prevention interventions that can be combined quickly and easily to create comprehensive evidence-based prevention services. Combining interrelated prevention services rather than delivering such services independently provides two critical benefits:

- Provides prevention service providers with greater flexibility when responding to changing disease epidemics or policy/political priorities by allowing them to build upon existing program infrastructures (e.g., human, information technology, financial) of multiple programs; and

- Lowers the total cost of service provision.

The U.S. GAO defines service integration as being either system-oriented or service-oriented.[27] A system-oriented service integration is one in which agencies attempt to create new integrated programs and structures for the provision of new services. A service-oriented integration is one in which agencies try only to provide persons with integrated services at a common setting, while maintaining their own programs and structures.

Service integration has two main goals:

- To make it easier for persons to access needed services by providing them with a single point of entry (such as a community health center in an inner-city area that also provides services such as welfare assistance, economic development assistance, and adult education); and

- To increase staff members' knowledge about available resources that are shared with other programs or agencies, and thereby minimize duplication of services while allowing each program or agency to continue specializing in its own area of expertise.

Service integration provides persons with seamless services from multiple programs or areas within programs without repeated registration procedures, waiting periods, or other administrative barriers.

A Framework for Service Integration

NCHHSTP proposes three levels of service integration at the client–provider interface (see examples in Table 2). The PCSI levels of integration incorporate a platform of standards that allows jurisdictions to (1) increase efficiency and reduce redundancy and missed opportunities for prevention and treatment by integrating services when appropriate; (2) increase flexibility of responses to evolving epidemics by enabling partners to adapt, implement structural/system changes, update policies, and modify integrated services; and (3) increase control over their operations by using local information derived from surveillance, program data, and key performance indicators.

- Level 1: Nonintegrated Services: Prevention services that are completely separate or not integrated at the point of client care (e.g., single-point testing for HIV only, other STDs only, or TB only).

- Level 2: Core Integrated Services: A basic package of services that integrates two or more CDC-recommended HIV/AIDS, viral hepatitis, STD and TB prevention, screening, testing, or treatment services into clinical care.

NCHHSTP currently recommends that, at a minimum, core integrated services include routine HIV testing consistent with the 2006 CDC *Revised Recommendations for HIV testing of Adults, Adolescents, and Pregnant Women in Health-Care Settings;*[14] chlamydia screening for women younger than 26 years of age;[29] provision of hepatitis B vaccination in clinical, nonclinical (e.g., outreach)[30] and correctional settings;[31] documented and tracked referrals to specialized services upon request or as indicated; and provision of health information on HIV, other STDs, viral hepatitis, and TB, including locations of local testing and treatment services.

Level 2 integrated services are based on published CDC recommendations. In addition to disease-specific recommendations such as those listed above, providers should review CDC recommendations by population and service delivery site to identify other appropriate Level 2 integration activities. Examples of typical Level 2 integrated services include TB clinics in which routine HIV testing is provided to persons with latent and active TB and their contacts; STD clinics that offer routine HIV testing and hepatitis B vaccination to all persons seeking care; emergency departments that routinely offer opt-out HIV testing to all newly admitted patients; and family-planning services that offer routine chlamydia screening to all women younger than 26 years.

- Level 3: Expanded Integrated Services: A comprehensive package of best and promising evidence-based practice of HIV/AIDS, viral hepatitis, STD, and TB prevention, screening, or treatment services that are integrated into general health and social services. Although the range of expanded integrated services may vary greatly, they may include the following examples as appropriate:

  - Comprehensive HIV/AIDS, viral hepatitis, STD and TB screening, diagnosis, and treatment services, with referral to specialized services and primary care, if required;

  - Comprehensive sexual and reproductive health and behavioral risk assessment, including assessment of drug use, mental health, and risk of intimate partner violence;

- Comprehensive reproductive health services, including pregnancy testing and contraceptive services;

- Specialized or social services, such as social case management and housing, drug addiction counseling, and mental health services;

- Health education and provision of targeted risk-reduction information; and

- Referral to other specialized and prevention services (e.g., behavioral interventions to help reduce or eliminate high-risk behaviors), as indicated.

Examples of Level 3 integrated services include services provided by many community health centers; lesbian, gay, bisexual, transgender (LGBT) health centers; and some comprehensive HIV/AIDS care providers, such as routine screening for alcohol or substance abuse at intake.

Expanded integrated services are based on best and promising evidence-based practices where CDC guidelines, standards, or recommendations may or may not exist.

Table 2. Program Collaboration and Service Integration Levels for NCHHSTP Prevention Services.		
Level of Integration	**Definition**	**Examples/ Features(s)**
Nonintegrated Services (Level 1)	Prevention, treatment, or care services provided for a single condition (HIV/AIDS, viral hepatitis, STD, or TB) by a single program.	• Persons are provided tests or services for a single condition at the point of access (e.g., HIV testing site). • Referral to allied prevention services may or may not be provided. • Health information on HIV/AIDS, STD, viral hepatitis, and TB, including locations of local services, may or may not be readily available.
Core Integrated Services (Level 2)	Integration of two or more CDC-recommended prevention, treatment or care services across HIV/AIDS, STD, viral hepatitis, or TB infections.	• Services that integrate routine HIV screening into clinical care (e.g., local health departments, TB clinics, emergency departments, STD clinics) are provided. • Routine screening is conducted for TB and STDs, and hepatitis A and B immunization provided for persons who are HIV positive. • Integrated population and individual risk factor assessment data are systematically collected each time a person receives health services to prevent missed opportunities for prevention.
Expanded Integrated Services (Level 3)	Integration of multiple prevention, treatment, and care services for HIV/AIDS, viral hepatitis, STD, and TB into general health and social services. CDC guidelines, standards, or recommendations for the delivery of these services may or may not exist.	• Comprehensive HIV/AIDS, viral hepatitis, STD, TB screening, diagnosis, treatment, and social services are offered in clinical or community health settings (i.e., community health centers, LGBT health centers). • Social services and case management are used to address housing needs, Medicaid problems, and/or drug addiction among persons diagnosed with HIV/AIDS, viral hepatitis, STD, and TB.

Note: Healthcare settings refer to all settings where healthcare providers work.

The proposed PCSI levels-of-integration framework makes it possible to identify, describe, and measure the types of integrated services provided within specific jurisdictions and settings. Components within each level may be expected to change as the epidemiology of diseases in various subpopulations evolves, new technologies are developed, new interventions become available and CDC guidelines are revised.

The framework is designed to be flexible enough to allow the combination and implementation of key prevention services in any healthcare setting: clinical, nonclinical, outreach, and behavioral intervention. Regardless of the level of integration, agencies receiving NCHHSTP funds will be expected to deliver high-quality prevention services and to report on certain integration performance indicators. Ongoing local evaluation of the impact of PCSI on service delivery and identification of best PCSI practices will be necessary.

Applying the PCSI Levels-of-Integration Framework to Service-Provision Settings

The provision of integrated services is particularly important in certain settings where high rates of infection are found. During the 2007 external consultation described previously, a limited number of settings were used to demonstrate the utility of applying the levels of integration to basic and expanded service delivery. Examples of how the levels of integration could be applied are shown in Tables 3 and 4. The levels of integration can also be applied in other settings where the integration of clinical and prevention services is important, such as substance abuse treatment centers and community health centers, as well as in nonclinical settings like outreach, behavioral intervention and other prevention programs.

The levels-of-integration framework can be applied in various settings. It allows for flexibility in addressing local conditions and for establishing baseline information for measuring progress. By using this framework, organizations can better differentiate themselves by how they conduct prevention activities, not merely by what prevention services they offer. Application of this framework should translate into greater client satisfaction, improved return on prevention investments and greater control over prevention services offered.

Table 3. Application of the Levels of Integration Framework in an STD, TB, Correctional Institution or HIV Setting for Core Service Integration (Level 2).

Core Service Integration (Level 2)	STD Clinical Setting	TB Clinical Setting	Correctional Institution	HIV Clinical Setting
Examples of Activities	All patients seeking treatment for STDs are screened routinely for HIV during each visit for a new concern, regardless of whether the patient is known or suspected to have specific behaviors for HIV infection. STD clinics routinely offer HBV vaccination as recommended to patients. Referrals to care for HIV-positive persons are documented and tracked. Partner services are offered to HIV-positive persons.	All patients who have confirmed or suspected TB are screened for HIV infection. Referrals to care for HIV-positive persons are documented and tracked.	Routine HIV testing, TB screening, and vaccination for viral hepatitis A and B (HAV/HBV) are provided. HCV testing is done. Inmates are referred to HIV clinical services during and after their incarceration, and their progress is tracked.	TB, syphilis, chlamydia, and gonorrhea screening is conducted for newly diagnosed HIV-positive persons.[32] HBV immunization and HCV testing are provided for all patients. Ongoing, routine assessment of risk behaviors and at least annual screening are done for syphilis and other STDs. Partner services are offered to HIV-positive persons.
Example Indicators	Percentage of persons treated for an STD who are tested for HIV infection. Percentage of eligible persons receiving HBV vaccination.	Percentage of persons treated for TB who are tested for HIV infection. Percentage of persons with newly diagnosed HIV/TB co-infection who are referred and linked to quality HIV care.	Percentage of inmates screened for HIV, TB, and viral hepatitis. Number of inmates diagnosed with syphilis, chlamydia and/or gonorrhea. Percentage of inmates receiving HAV/HBV vaccination. Percentage of tested inmates who test positive for HIV, TB, or viral hepatitis.	Percentage of HIV-positive persons who are screened for TB, syphilis, chlamydia, and/or gonorrhea. Percentage of HIV-positive persons offered partner services.

Table 4. Application of the Levels-of-Integration Framework in an STD, TB, Correctional Institution, or HIV Setting for Expanded Service Integration (Level 3).

Expanded Service Integration (Level 3)	STD Clinical Setting	TB Clinical Setting	Correctional Institution	HIV Clinical Setting
Example of Activities	Persons at high risk are recruited and referred to HIV prevention behavioral interventions.	Comprehensive HIV, STD, and viral hepatitis prevention services, as well as reproductive, drug/alcohol/mental, and health risk assessment and services are provided for TB patients. Case management for housing/drug/alcohol/mental health and other services is provided.	Comprehensive HIV, STD, and viral hepatitis prevention services as well as reproductive, drug/alcohol/mental counseling, and health risk assessment and services are provided for TB patients. Case management for housing/drug/alcohol/mental health and discharge planning is provided to ensure that inmates receive appropriate follow-up care in the community. Routine syphilis, chlamydia and gonorrhea screening is provided.	Comprehensive TB, STD, and viral hepatitis prevention services as well as partner services, behavioral interventions, reproductive, drug/alcohol/mental, and health risk assessment are provided.
Example Indicators	Percentage of persons at high risk for HIV infection who are enrolled into HIV behavioral interventions.	Percentage of homeless persons being treated for TB who receive case management for social services.	Percentage of inmates with diagnosed HIV, syphilis, chlamydia, gonorrhea, TB, or viral hepatitis who receive comprehensive discharge planning and continued care.	Percentage of high-risk persons found to have TB, STD, or viral hepatitis infection.

PUBLIC HEALTH AND RELATED PREVENTION SERVICES

Program Collaboration and Service Integration has implications for key areas in public health and related prevention services. Publicly funded local, state and national partners should ensure that barriers are adequately addressed and policies and procedures are in place to facilitate collaboration across HIV/AIDS, viral hepatitis, other STDs and TB programs at multiple levels and coordinate the delivery of integrated services at the client level, where these services intersect.

Public Health Services

Surveillance

Public health surveillance may be defined as the ongoing systematic collection, analysis, and interpretation of data for use in the planning, implementation and evaluation of public health practice.[33] Although the fundamental activities of surveillance are data collection, analysis and dissemination, the true value of surveillance is measured through its impetus for public health action and impact on public health practice.[34]

For example, surveillance data can provide a more complete picture of the population of persons newly diagnosed in the public and private sectors who are in need of partner services for HIV or STD. The integration of HIV/AIDS, viral hepatitis, STD and TB surveillance data will be important in (1) enhancing the quality of surveillance data across programs; (2) understanding how these diseases overlap geographically, within population subgroups, or within groups engaging in specified high-risk behaviors; and (3) understanding how these overlaps might affect the effectiveness and efficiency of public health programs.[34] Compatibility of data elements and interoperable surveillance systems greatly increase the ability to develop a comprehensive view of surveillance data, syndemics, and the populations at risk.

NCHHSTP recognizes that systems duplication and inefficiencies most often impact programs at the local and state levels, where the burden is made more difficult by having completely separate reporting systems for each disease, i.e., Tuberculosis Information Management System (TIMS), Sexually Transmitted Disease Management Information System (STD*MIS), Enhanced HIV/AIDS Reporting System (eHARS), and the National Electronic Disease Surveillance System (NEDSS) for viral hepatitis. During the last decade, numerous advances have occurred in how health information is collected (e.g., name-based reporting), managed, and analyzed. Much of the information needed for disease surveillance is now stored in electronic formats, creating opportunities for automation of disease reporting and surveillance tasks—many of which are currently labor-intensive, paper-based processes.

The true value of surveillance is measured through its impetus for public health action and impact on public health practice.

Surveillance integration could be facilitated by a commitment to minimizing the barriers to data sharing that currently exist and by providing incentives for the creation of more comprehensive surveillance systems. As an initial step, NCHHSTP is working to develop common confidentiality and security standards across its national programs and across state, and local health programs. NCHHSTP hopes that this effort will provide data sharing standards for some programs that have never had them, while clarifying appropriate levels of access to facilitate the two-way sharing of data by programs that have been reluctant to do so in the past. NCHHSTP is also committed to developing a shared vision and strategy for promoting integrated surveillance in the intermediate term—a strategy that will complement and take advantage of the opportunities created through healthcare reform and modernization of health information technologies.

Training and Workforce Development

Successful implementation of PCSI will require ongoing training and support for public health prevention workers, including clinicians, in a variety of healthcare and community-based settings over sustained periods.

> Clinical providers will need to be trained in integrated risk assessment, prevention counseling, and provision of prevention services and referrals.

> Staff in many community-based organizations will need to be trained in delivering more holistic clinical, immunization and prevention services and referrals.

> Health department personnel and federal field and headquarters staff will need to be trained in service-delivery integration and integrated data management and will need to be provided with opportunities to work across programs.

For most staff members, additional skill development will be important because many have been trained in or have worked in only one or two areas. For example, HIV-prevention workers will need to become knowledgeable about STD, viral hepatitis, and TB testing, treatment, and vaccination services, while clinicians will need to become more knowledgeable about the range of available behavioral prevention services that can be incorporated into clinical care or provided through referrals.

All NCHHSTP programs provide training and technical assistance on a variety of topics. In addition, NCHHSTP encourages state and local programs to allow prevention workers to broaden their public health expertise through training outside the scope of their current positions. As more programs implement PCSI and make progress in appropriate integration of services, training across program lines will become increasingly important for more workers. NCHHSTP will ensure cross-program support of CDC headquarters staff, field staff and local health department staff, when justified and appropriate.

Laboratory Services

Laboratory services are critical for the diagnosis, clinical management, and surveillance of communicable diseases. In most instances, laboratory diagnostic services are provided in response to requests from healthcare providers. As service integration becomes a dominant programmatic approach to patient care, a demand for integrated laboratory services will naturally follow. Laboratory workflow, ordering and procurement systems, and data-reporting systems will need to be redesigned to accommodate these demands. A laboratory relational diagram can be found in Appendix 2. These challenges will be unique from jurisdiction to jurisdiction, and each should examine all areas of their approach to diagnostic support and communication between laboratories and programs.

Rapid point-of-care tests allow healthcare providers to make more timely diagnoses and to offer services in nonclinical and outreach settings while patients await preliminary test results. Point-of-care test results are also frequently reported back to programs to inform them of presumptive diagnoses. However, laboratory testing remains the mainstay for confirmatory diagnoses. With the growing popularity of point-of-care and combination testing for multiple diseases, more sophisticated testing algorithms need to be developed. These algorithms will have significant bearing on the accuracy of diagnoses and the clinical management of patients. Development of bridging algorithms to establish decision points for transitioning between point-of-care and laboratory-based diagnostic tests might be considered as jurisdictions undertake large-scale implementation of new on-site diagnostic approaches.

Laboratory services are critical for the diagnosis, clinical management, and surveillance of communicable diseases.

Combination point-of-care testing may be one mechanism for better integration of clinical services. However, the availability of point-of-care diagnostic tests currently varies for different diseases, and an integrated diagnostic algorithm will most certainly involve a combination of point-of-care and laboratory-based testing. Public health laboratories will therefore have important roles in determining how best to use such testing and should work closely with programmatic staff at all levels to help guide appropriate testing approaches. Public health laboratories can also provide a vital quality assurance component to monitor the reliability and accuracy of point-of-care testing. Systems to evaluate the performance of these tests under various settings and in low-incidence disease areas will need to be established to determine the limitations of their use.

Combination point-of-care testing may be one mechanism for better integration of clinical services.

With the increasing contribution of high-throughput diagnostic services provided by commercial laboratories, many public health laboratories are struggling to control costs and maintain a necessary level of preparedness. Therefore, it is even more vital that public health laboratory managers discuss integrated approaches with programmatic leadership and carefully consider how to process, store, and distribute diagnostic specimens most efficiently. In some instances, distribution might be simplified by having sample processing and some diagnostic testing performed at a single laboratory. However, diagnostic specimens may have to be routed to multiple laboratories to accomplish the various diagnostic tests requested as part of an integrated approach to services. Therefore, public health laboratories should anticipate increased costs associated with the potential increased demand for diagnostic services under an integrated approach to service delivery. The increases in costs associated with doing more tests could be partially offset with a thorough assessment of factors contributing to the increased costs.

Test results from multiple laboratories will require increased attention, although the complexity of such reporting should be reduced by progress toward general electronic reporting of laboratory data. In the meantime, central aspects of data sharing among healthcare providers, state and local health departments, and epidemiologic or surveillance programs must be coordinated. Regular communication and planning between laboratories and programs might greatly decrease redundancies in testing and reporting. Jurisdictional consensus around this issue is necessary, and coordination of existing laboratory information systems might require focused effort and resources. In some instances, data will also have to be shared with partner services for use in public health action and program assessment activities. Appropriately routing and sharing diagnostic results while maintaining patient confidentiality will require cooperation among the various programs involved.

Maintaining the infrastructure of public health laboratories and appropriate training of laboratory workers are essential to NCHHSTP's PCSI efforts. The multiple resource streams available to public health laboratories may have to be considered, especially as programmatic outreach to affected populations shifts with time. Training laboratory workers across several diagnostic areas may be required. Partnerships and collaboration between NCHHSTP and outside laboratories will continue to be critical for maintaining vital diagnostic services and accurate surveillance.

Communication

NCHHSTP will continue working on collaboration and service integration, share best practices, and exchange ideas for research or implementation by facilitating widespread dialogue on PCSI at national conferences and with the Advisory Council for the Elimination of Tuberculosis (ACET), CDC Board of Scientific Counselors (BSC), Health Resources and Services Administration (HRSA), CDC/HRSA Advisory Committee (CHAC), Office of Population Affairs (OPA), Substance Abuse and Mental Health Services Administration (SAMHSA), and national professional organizations, such as the Association of Public Health Laboratories (APHL), the Association of State and Territorial Health Officials (ASTHO), the National Alliance of State and Territorial AIDS Directors (NASTAD), the National Association of Community Health Centers (NACHC), the National Association of County and City Health Officials (NACCHO), the National Coalition of STD Directors (NCSD), the National Tuberculosis Controllers Association (NTCA), and the Urban Coalition of HIV/AIDS Prevention Services (UCHAPS).

Related Prevention Services

Partner Services

Partner services and contact tracing have been important public health tools in the United States for decades. Although partner services is often associated with STDs, including HIV, similar methods of investigation and contact tracing have been used by TB control programs for years and have more recently been employed to identify those in contact with persons infected with severe acute respiratory syndrome (SARS), monkeypox, and rabies.[35] Regardless of the pathogen or its routes of transmission, the goals of partner services and contact tracing are to identify others who may have been exposed; offer and provide testing, treatment, and prevention services; and prevent further disease exposure or transmission.

Initial variations in how partner services for STDs and HIV were conducted led to different and confusing program requirements and the use of different data-collection tools, performance metrics, guidance documents, and training programs. As a result, exposed partners were often not being identified as quickly as they should be, their identification often required more than one interview, and they often were not being offered appropriate services.

In 2007, NCHHSTP's Division of STD Prevention and Division of HIV/AIDS Prevention jointly developed a harmonized and integrated patient-interview record. In 2008, integrated recommendations on partner services for HIV infection, syphilis, gonorrhea,

Regardless of the pathogen or its routes of transmission, the goals of partner services and contact tracing are to

- *identify others who may have been exposed.*
- *offer and provide testing, treatment, and prevention services.*
- *prevent further disease exposure or transmission.*

and chlamydia infection were released with appropriate training to follow.[36] As NCHHSTP continues its PCSI activities, partner services programs should be able to demonstrate, through monitoring and evaluation, the extent to which their services are being provided in accordance with the new recommendations. State and local programs are encouraged to work with their counterparts at NCHHSTP to integrate partner services at the local level.

Behavioral Interventions

For the infectious diseases within NCHHSTP's purview, prevention services other than clinical play a critical role at the individual and community levels. At the individual level, health education, health promotion and risk-reduction interventions are important to keeping at-risk individuals from acquiring disease in the first place. Beyond individual level interventions, network interventions aim to affect subpopulations by identifying and intervening within a social network, while community-level and structural interventions provide greater saturation and intervention coverage and are aimed at altering community norms or creating public health policies that alter the surrounding environment.

For persons who acquire an infectious disease, prevention services are important in reducing risky behavior and transmission of disease, promoting treatment adherence, and offering clinical and prevention services to other potentially exposed individuals.

Though individual and group interventions are important mechanisms for reaching individuals at high risk, there are insufficient resources to scale these interventions to reach population-level impact in most jurisdictions. Individually based interventions may be more effective for individual participants, particularly those at high risk, but they have limited population coverage.[37] In contrast, population-based efforts target a large percentage of the population, but they typically have lower levels of individual-based effectiveness. However, small changes at the population level can lead to large effects on disease risk.[38]

Both individual- and population-level interventions are important; thus a multilevel approach to prevention services is desirable. The focus of PCSI is on greater consistency of integrated messages within interventions and across interventions. By linking interventions, greater consistency can eventually be achieved in intervention messages, support and follow-up.

Health Education and Messaging

In addition to integrated services, providers should select appropriate, comprehensive prevention messages for the populations they serve. Providing accurate, timely and useful health information to individuals and communities is critical to NCHHSTP's prevention efforts. Bundling and integrating health messages to individuals and subpopulations with overlapping risks for multiple infections may help promote health equity and address the needs of individuals and communities in a more holistic, influential, and cost-effective way. Given that the populations most affected by HIV, viral hepatitis, and other STDs are similar (e.g., men who have sex with men and African Americans), greater emphasis on integrating messages and developing social marketing campaigns that encourage appropriate testing and treatment for all these diseases as well as the use of other prevention services are needed. Such PCSI efforts should occur at all stages of health communication efforts (e.g., qualitative and quantitative research, implementation and scale-up and evaluation).

State and local programs are encouraged to work with their counterparts at NCHHSTP to integrate partner services at the local level.

The focus of PCSI is on greater consistency of integrated messages within interventions and across interventions.

Bundling and integrating health messages to individuals and subpopulations with overlapping risks for multiple infections may help promote health equity.

MONITORING AND EVALUATION

NCHHSTP is committed to the ongoing monitoring and evaluation of PCSI and expects similar commitment from the agencies that it funds. NCHHSTP has two goals related to PCSI evaluation:

- To estimate the number and type of PCSI activities among grantees; and

- To monitor internal NCHHSTP progress on PCSI-related activities and the effect of these activities on programs and at the point of service delivery.

NCHHSTP intends to use PCSI monitoring and evaluation information to track progress toward goals and objectives, identify and address the primary barriers that prevent increased or improved PCSI, and identify processes and practices within and outside of NCHHSTP that are particularly effective for promoting PCSI. PCSI monitoring and evaluation information will assist NCHHSTP leadership in making mid-course corrections to current activities and planning new activities that have the most promise.

NCHHSTP has developed an evaluation plan for its PCSI activities in consultation with key stakeholders within CDC and external national professional associations. The plan includes a logic model describing NCHHSTP PCSI activities and their intended outcomes (Appendix 3), and the primary evaluation questions, indicators, and data sources to track key national-level processes and outcomes[39] (available at www.cdc.gov/nchhstp/programintegration).

The logic model presented in Appendix 3 depicts examples of NCHHSTP's primary PCSI-related activities, the intended outcomes of those activities, and the pathways through which these activities are to produce the intended outcomes. The logic model articulates both shorter- and longer-term intended outcomes and distinguishes between intended outcomes for grantees and those related to internal functions within the Center. Evaluation questions and related indicators, as well as existing data sources, are described in the plan.

Monitoring and evaluation are key components of the successful implementation of PCSI, as these activities directly relate to the Five Principles of Effective PCSI. Monitoring and evaluation are the tools used to assess appropriateness, effectiveness, acceptability and the mechanism by which programs achieve flexibility and accountability. The information gleaned from ongoing monitoring and evaluation helps programs identify what is working, what needs adjustment, and how to refine activities to achieve optimal results; thus empowering programs to make changes that improve health outcomes and reduce cost. NCHHSTP recommends that programs continually obtain input on proposed and planned changes, and then assess the effectiveness and consequences (intended or unintended) resulting from changes in policies and procedures on programs, providers and clients.

PCSI monitoring and evaluation involves the use of evaluation questions, process measures, and performance indicators. Process measures for program functions would be specific to jurisdictions and dependent on locally identified strategies. Performance indicators help show the degree to which program targets have been achieved. Process measures and performance indicators allow programs to compare actual outcomes with anticipated outcomes, and to determine whether an activity is on schedule and is being implemented as planned. Previous sections of this white paper provide examples of

PCSI monitoring and evaluation information will assist leadership in planning new activities that have the most promise.

Monitoring and evaluation are key components of the successful implementation of PCSI.

collaboration activities with corresponding process measures (Table 1) and service integration with corresponding indicators (Tables 3,4).

Multiple performance indicators based on health service delivery data are already collected by local jurisdictions or may be readily captured by existing information-management systems at the local level. Others may need to be collected through tailored studies or audits within clinical settings. Key characteristics of these performance indicators include their validity (ability to monitor actual performance); their adaptability (ability to identify and adjust to changes in clinical activity levels, disease epidemiology, or demographic groups most affected by diseases); and their usefulness in quality-assurance assessments.

Programs should monitor effectiveness, yield and outputs resulting from service integration and consider the following suggested evaluation questions:

a. To what extent has program collaboration increased across disease areas within jurisdictions? What barriers to collaboration remain?

b. What is the level of service integration across disease areas at the point of service delivery?

c. What is the impact of PCSI on health outcomes? Are there reductions in HIV-associated TB, STD-related HIV infections, or concurrent transmission of HIV, viral hepatitis and sexually transmitted diseases?

d. How has service integration changed over time? What barriers to service integration remain? What unintended effects has PCSI had on the delivery of HIV, viral hepatitis, STD, and TB services?

CDC's Framework for Program Evaluation in Public Health states that "Because categorical strategies cannot succeed in isolation, public health professionals working across program areas must collaborate in evaluating their combined influence on program changes and service integration to improve health in the community."[40] This framework provides a detailed description of how to approach monitoring and evaluation activities.

Operational Research

Two of the five principles of PCSI, effectiveness and acceptability, are particularly relevant for operational research. Participants in the 2007 external consultation concerning NCHHSTP's PCSI efforts recommended that NCHHSTP develop an operational research and evaluation agenda for PCSI to assess whether integrated services are efficient, effective and acceptable to patients and providers and to identify best and promising PCSI practices.

Pursuant to establishing a PCSI research agenda, NCHHSTP described its preliminary PCSI plans to the Board of Scientific Counselors (BSC) of CDC's Coordinating Center for Infectious Diseases (CCID), an external advisory group of scientists that meets regularly to review the activities of and provide advice to NCHHSTP and the other centers within CCID. Following a BSC meeting on May 6, 2008, the Board recommended that NCHHSTP establish three overarching PCSI research priorities: evaluation of the effectiveness of integration, operational research on integration, and research on integrated health communication. NCHHSTP is adopting the recommendations of the BSC. The three research priorities are described in detail in Appendix 4.

TOWARD IMPLEMENTATION

CDC recognizes that many state and local programs have a rich history of productive collaboration on a variety of important programs and activities. NCHHSTP units have also engaged increasingly in cross-division and cross-program communication and coordination. Acknowledging and building upon these collaborations will be crucial to the success of NCHHSTP's additional PCSI efforts.

PCSI Strategic Priorities

Participants in the PCSI consultation meeting in 2007 generally agreed that NCHHSTP should begin by focusing on three key areas of its PCSI efforts:

- Integrated surveillance
- Integrated programming
- Integrated training

However, NCHHSTP's PCSI activities will not be limited to these three areas and programs should continue to pursue collaboration and integration in all activities while following the principles for effective PCSI: appropriateness, effectiveness, flexibility, accountability and acceptability.

Integrated Surveillance

NCHHSTP recognizes the importance of supporting integrated surveillance, data harmonization, and data sharing. NCHHSTP will actively support opportunities to demonstrate the feasibility and acceptability of surveillance integration efforts and the added value of integrated surveillance and program data.

Potential priority areas include:

- Documenting current business practices related to integrated electronic laboratory reporting;
- Developing economic cost/benefit analyses to guide future development of integrated surveillance;
- Drafting protocols for integrated confidentiality standards;
- Developing an integrated epidemiologic profile for HIV/AIDS, viral hepatitis, STD, and TB;
- Conducting electronic matching of case surveillance registries;
- Assessing laboratory information systems and electronic sharing of diagnostic results; and
- Evaluating the level of service integration in prevention service settings.

NCHHSTP will seek to improve collaboration in surveillance by reducing barriers to sharing and using surveillance data while maintaining or improving systems that protect patient confidentiality.

PCSI Strategic Priorities

- *Integrated Surveillance*
- *Integrated Program*
- *Integrated Training*

Integrated Programming

NCHHSTP is committed to finding opportunities to increase flexibility in the use of funds and facilitate collaboration among programs at multiple levels. Core funding opportunity announcements (FOAs) will be cataloged, and new FOAs will include more explicit language on how funds may be used to support PCSI. NCHHSTP divisions will collaborate on the development of future FOAs so that the purpose of funding, key activities and evaluation criteria reflect support for collaborative work and integrated services. State and local jurisdictions and other entities that distribute funds should replicate NCHHSTP's integrated approach in their funding streams. Funding entities should identify key funding announcements and as existing contracts and grants expire, work collaboratively on the development of request for proposals (RFPs) that foster appropriate collaboration and service integration among grantees. Funding entities must ensure that funds are always used as they are intended by Congress, CDC, or other principal funder. Generally, it is justifiable and appropriate to structure FOAs so that funds can be used for activities that have a direct impact on the primary disease (e.g., the presence of an STD increases the likelihood of HIV transmission or identifying the presence of an STD can directly improve HIV prevention).

Integrated Training

NCHHSTP will support integrated training and capacity building. By working with its training branches and funded training partners existing curricula will be reviewed for integration opportunities and to develop appropriate integrated training.

Other NCHHSTP Strategic Commitments to PCSI

NCHHSTP will seek to enhance collaboration with its external partners, including other federal agencies, state and local health departments, community-based organizations and professional organizations through formal and informal mechanisms. To facilitate widespread dialogue on PCSI, NCHHSTP will ensure continued PCSI presentations, discussions and sharing of best practices at national prevention conferences and key meetings with national professional organizations.

NCHHSTP will continue to develop and publish integrated program guidelines and recommendations for providing services to persons who have or are at risk for more than one disease. The Recommendations for Partner Services Programs for HIV Infection, Syphilis, Gonorrhea, and Chlamydial Infection[36] are exemplary and highlight the importance of program collaboration and service integration in the provision of partner services. NCHHSTP is committed to this integrated approach and to supporting and expanding similar opportunities for integration of services.

NCHHSTP is committed to an integrated and holistic approach to partner services and encourages local STD, HIV/AIDS, and surveillance programs to work with their counterparts at NCHHSTP to integrate partner services at the local level.

NCHHSTP will design and evaluate integrated health communication that focus on populations rather than diseases. As part of this effort, NCHHSTP will develop and promote comprehensive HIV/AIDS/viral hepatitis/STD prevention messages about sexual risks, particularly when developing messages and behavioral interventions for populations at risk for multiple infections.

As existing contracts and grants expire, funders should work collaboratively on the development of RFPs that foster appropriate collaboration and service integration among grantees.

Funds should always be used as they are intended, by Congress, CDC, or other principal funder.

Other NCHHSTP Strategic Commitments

- *Partnerships*
- *Integrated guidelines and recommendations*
- *Partner services*
- *Integrated health communication*
- *Evaluation and research*

NCHHSTP will continue to support research needed to demonstrate how collaboration and service integration can improve program effectiveness and health outcomes of persons served.

NCHHSTP will develop a plan for evaluating its PCSI activities and their impact on short- and long-term outcomes important to NCHHSTP and its grantees.

What Can State and Local Jurisdictions Do?

State and local jurisdictions receiving NCHHSTP funds, directly or indirectly, will be expected to deliver high-quality prevention services and to report on certain integration performance indicators. NCHHSTP will encourage their ongoing evaluation of PCSI's impact on service delivery and identification of best PCSI practices. The following are ways in which state and local programs can incorporate PCSI into their day-to-day operations and delivery of services:

- Adopt PCSI as a strategic imperative for your state, local health department, agency, clinic or unit. Then hold the organization accountable for PCSI adoption by identifying key PCSI priorities, assessing progress toward meeting PCSI goals, and reporting this progress on a regular basis (e.g., in annual reports).

- Obtain clear political commitment to PCSI and PCSI-related activities. Discuss identified barriers that prohibit collaboration or integrated service delivery and the proposed improvements with key constituents. Develop mutually beneficial plans that reduce operational barriers to PCSI, and obtain input on the highest priorities for action. Continually obtain input on proposed and planned changes, and assess the effectiveness and consequences (intended or unintended) resulting from changes in policies and procedures on programs, providers and clients.

- Identify an appropriate senior organizational leader to be a PCSI "champion," and create a PCSI coalition. This coalition will be responsible for working across the organization to raise awareness about PCSI, identify PCSI opportunities, articulate priorities for implementation, facilitate collaboration and/or service integrations, and evaluate PCSI progress. Support a coalition of committed local colleagues and sponsor forums (e.g., PCSI workgroup, journal clubs, seminars, integrated workgroups) within the organization to discuss PCSI, identify priorities for and barriers to PCSI implementation, disseminate best practices, and celebrate successful implementations of PCSI.

- Assess and articulate how PCSI can improve local service delivery. Use the best available evidence to understand the intersections and overlaps apparent in HIV/AIDS, viral hepatitis, STD and TB epidemics among populations in your jurisdiction or agency's care, and to what extent integrated services are offered and collaborations are currently occurring to address these. Articulate the ways in which an integrated approach to preventing these diseases would be an improvement over a disease-specific approach that is currently used. Describe the needed changes in policies, procedures and methods to integrate service delivery. Share talking points and key resources with colleagues, grantees and local communities.

- Support evidence-based practices in the adoption of PCSI, and evaluate PCSI's impact on behavioral and health outcomes. Commit to disseminating lessons learned about PCSI in scientific journals, at conferences and in other appropriate venues.

Develop mutually beneficial plans that reduce operational barriers to PCSI.

Use the best available evidence to understand the intersections and overlaps apparent in HIV/AIDS, viral hepatitis, STD, and TB epidemics among populations in your jurisdiction.

CONCLUSIONS

NCHHSTP and its prevention partners will continue to seek ways to improve collaboration in the delivery of holistic prevention services to those in need. Evolving epidemiology, common risk behaviors, similar modes of transmission, concurrent disease interactions, and significant opportunities to improve services while eliminating duplication require PCSI adoption. PCSI is an important tool that can help give programs enhanced flexibility, efficiency and control in the delivery of those services.

CDC acknowledges the tremendous work that many of its partners have done in collaborating and integrating services and hopes to build upon their accomplishments through a more systematic approach to PCSI. CDC believes that by using the PCSI principles of effectiveness described in this paper, programs can deliver more comprehensive integrated services and thereby identify and treat disease more effectively and improve the behavioral and health outcomes of the persons they serve.

About NCHHSTP

NCHHSTP is responsible for public health surveillance, prevention research and programs to prevent and control HIV infection, AIDS, viral hepatitis, other sexually transmitted diseases and tuberculosis. NCHHSTP works in collaboration with governmental and nongovernmental partners at community, state, national and international levels, applying well-integrated multidisciplinary programs of research, surveillance, technical assistance and evaluation.

PCSI is an important tool that can help give programs enhanced flexibility, efficiency and control in the delivery of holistic prevention services.

For additional information on PCSI and PCSI levels of integration, visit the NCHHSTP Web site (http://www.cdc.gov/nchhstp) or contact NCHHSTP at pcsi@cdc.gov or call 404-639-8009.

REFERENCES

1. Frieden TR, Das-Douglas M, Kellerman SE, Henning KJ. Applying public health principles to the HIV epidemic. N Engl J Med 2005;353:2397–2402.

2. Fox Fields H. The Integration of HIV/AIDS, STD, and TB prevention and control programs. Washington, DC: Association of State and Territorial Health Officials; 1998.

3. Wohlfeiler D. STD/HIV Prevention integration. National Alliance of State and Territorial AIDS Directors and National Coalition of STD Directors and the HIV/STD Work Group; June 2002. Available at: http://www.ihs.gov/medicalprograms/hivaids/docs/STDHIVIntegration.pdf.

4. Lush L. Service integration: an overview of policy developments. Int Fam Plan Perspect 2002;28:71–76.

5. Jourden J, Etkind P. Enhancing HIV/AIDS and STD prevention through program integration. Public Health Rep 2004;119:4–11.

6. Meyerson B. Policy and program coordination: a shared challenge with miles yet to go. Public Health Rep 2004;119:2–3.

7. CDC. HIV prevention through early detection and treatment of other sexually transmitted diseases—United States. MMWR 1998;47(No. RR-12):1–24.

8. Milstein B. Introduction to the Syndemics Prevention Network. Atlanta, GA: Centers for Disease Control and Prevention; 2002. Available at: http://www.cdc.gov/syndemics/.

9. Buffington J, Jones TS. Integrating viral hepatitis prevention into public health programs serving people at high risk for infection: good public health. Public Health Rep 2007;122(Suppl 2):1–5.

10. Ward JW, Fenton KA. CDC and progress toward integration of HIV, STD, and viral hepatitis prevention. Public Health Rep 2007;122(Suppl 2):99–101.

11. Whiticar P. Liberti T. Advancing integration of HIV, STD, and viral hepatitis services: state perspectives. Public Health Rep 2007;122(Suppl 2):91–95.

12. Gunn RA, Lee, MA, Murry PA, Gilchick RA, Margolis HS. Hepatitis B vaccination of men who have sex with men attending an urban STD clinic: impact of an ongoing vaccination program, 1998–2003. Sex Transm Dis 2007;34:663–668.

13. Baldy LM, Urbas C, Harris JL, Jones TS, Reichert PE. Establishing a viral hepatitis control program: Florida's experience. Public Health Rep 2007;122(Suppl 2):24–31.

14. CDC. Revised recommendations for HIV testing of adults, adolescents, and pregnant women in health-care settings. MMWR 2006;55(No. RR-14):1–17.

15. Kresina TF, Hoffman K, Lubran R, Clark HW. Integrating hepatitis services into substance abuse treatment programs: new initiatives from SAMHSA. Public Health Rep 2007;122(Suppl 2):96–97.

16. Kendrick SR, Kroc KA, Withum D, Rydman RJ, Branson BM, Weinstein RA. Outcomes of offering rapid point-of-care HIV testing in a sexually transmitted disease clinic. J Acquir Immune Defic Syndr 2005;38:142–146.

17. Spielberg F, Branson BM, Goldbaum GM, et al. Overcoming barriers to HIV testing: preferences for new strategies among clients of a needle exchange, a sexually transmitted disease clinic, and sex venues for men who have sex with men. J Acquir Immune Defic Syndr 2003;32:318–328.

18. Gaydos CA. Nucleic acid amplification tests for gonorrhea and chlamydia: practice and applications. Infect Dis Clin North Am 2005;19:367–386.

19. CDC, NCHHSTP. NCHHSTP External consultation on program collaboration and service integration: Meeting report summary. Atlanta, GA: Centers for Disease Control and Prevention; 2007. Available at: http://www.cdc.gov/nchhstp/programintegration/docs/PCSImeetingreportwithcover11-26%20_2.pdf.

20. CDC, NCHHSTP. Program collaboration and service integration: enhancing the prevention and control of HIV/AIDS, viral hepatitis, STD, and TB in the United States, an NCHHSTP green paper. Atlanta, GA: Centers for Disease Control and Prevention; 2007. Available at: http://www.cdc.gov/nchhstp/programintegration/attachments/I-NCHHSTP-PCSIGreenPaper_508.pdf.

21. CDC. Essential components of a tuberculosis prevention and control program: recommendations of the Advisory Council for the Elimination of Tuberculosis. MMWR 1995;44(No. RR-11):1–16.

22. Hennessy RR, Weisfuse IB, Schlanger K. Does integrating viral hepatitis services into a public STD clinic attract injection drug users for care? Public Health Rep 2007;122 (Suppl 2):31–35.

23. Stopka TJ, Marshall C, Bluthenthal RN, Webb DS, Truax SR. HCV and HIV counseling and testing integration in California: an innovative approach to increase HIV counseling and testing rates. Public Health Rep 2007;122(Suppl 2):68–73.

24. Mattessich PW, Murray-Close M, Monsey BR. Collaboration: what makes it work. 2nd ed. St. Paul, MN: Amherst Wilder Foundation; 2001. Appendix A.

25. Chavis DM. Building community capacity to prevent violence through coalitions and partnerships. J Health Care Poor Underserved 1995;6:234–245.

26. Public Health Functions Steering Committee. Public health in America. Rockville, MD: US Department of Health and Human Services, Office of Disease Prevention and Health Promotion; 1994. Available at: http://www.health.gov/phfunctions/public.htm.

27. US General Accounting Office. Integrating human services: linking at-risk families with services more successful than system reform efforts. Washington, DC: US General Accounting Office; 1992. Report no. HRD-92-108. Available at: http://www.gao.gov.

28. Pindus N, Koralek R, Martinson K, Trutko J. Coordination and integration of welfare and workforce development systems. Washington, DC: Urban Institute; 2000. Available at: www.urban.org/UploadedPDF/coordination_FR.pdf.

29 CDC. Sexually transmitted diseases treatment guidelines, 2006. MMWR 2006;55 (No. RR-11):1–94.

30. CDC. A comprehensive immunization strategy to eliminate transmission of hepatitis B virus infection in the United States: recommendations of the Advisory Committee on Immunization Practices (ACIP). Part II: immunization of adults. MMWR 2006;55 (No. RR-16):1–25.

31. CDC. Prevention and control of infections with hepatitis viruses in correctional settings. MMWR 2003;52(No. RR-01):1–33.

32. CDC. Guidelines for prevention and treatment of opportunistic infections in HIV-infected adults and adolescents. MMWR 2009;58(No. RR-04):1–198.

33. Thacker SB. Historical development. In: Teutsch SM, Churchill RE, eds. Principles and practice of public health surveillance, 2nd ed. New York, NY: Oxford University Press; 2000.

34. Weinstock H, Douglas JM Jr, Fenton KA. Toward integration of STD, HIV, TB, and viral hepatitis surveillance. Public Health Rep. 2009; 124 (Suppl 2): 5-6.

35. Semaan S, Klovdahl A, Aral O. Protecting the privacy, confidentiality, relationships, and medical safety of sex partners in partner notification and management studies. J Research Admin 2004;35:39–53.

36. CDC. Recommendations for partner services programs for HIV infection, syphilis, gonorrhea, and chlamydial infection. MMWR 2008;57(No. RR-9):1–63.

37. Wohlfeiler D, Ellen JM. The limits of behavioral interventions for HIV prevention. In: Cohen L, Chavez V, Chehimi S, Cohen L, eds. Prevention is primary: strategies for community well-being. San Francisco, CA: Jossey-Bass; 2007. 329–347.

38. Emmons KM. Behavioral and social science contributions to the health of adults in the United States. In: Smedley BD, Syme SL, eds. Promoting health: intervention strategies from social and behavioral research. Washington, DC: National Academy Press; 2000. 254–321.

39. CDC, NCHHSTP. Program collaboration and service integration evaluation plan, 2009. Atlanta, GA. Centers for Disease Control and Prevention; 2009. Available at: www.cdc.gov/nchhstp/programintegration.

40. CDC. Framework for program evaluation in public health. MMWR 1999;48 (No. RR-11):1–40.

APPENDIX 1

Key Findings from the 2007 CDC PCSI Consultation Meeting

Top Priority Opportunities

1. Integrated Surveillance Efforts

    - Achieve leadership consensus for surveillance integration (agreement across geographic areas and programs, agreement on legal issues, partner engagement, and prioritizing integration).

    - Increase funding and resources for surveillance.

    - Build epidemiologic and surveillance capacity at the state and local level.

    - Develop common definitions of surveillance; harmonize data elements, formats, security and confidentiality standards across NCHHSTP programs.

2. Integrated Training Efforts

    - Increase workforce development and cross-training on NCHHSTP disease areas and prevention techniques for federal, state, and local public health staff.

    - Increase opportunities for shared training and education programs within NCHHSTP disease areas.

    - Develop and promote PCSI training and education to promote shared understanding and vision for state and local public health officials.

3. Integrated Funding Efforts

    - Develop and promote integrated NCHHSTP program announcements.

    - Promote and reward collaboration on NCHHSTP program announcements and post-award management at CDC.

    - Identify mechanisms and incentives for state and federal funding to support integration of NCHHSTP programs.

    - Allow flexibility of funds to accomplish state and local objectives.

    - Fund and support evaluation and operational research/evaluation on service delivery integration for NCHHSTP program areas.

Top Policy Improvements

Federal partners divided into two groups to prioritize the proposed policy improvements. The following are the policy improvements selected for the top three priorities:

1. Toward Integrated Surveillance

    - NCHHSTP divisions to develop internal and external work group on surveillance integration.

    - NCHHSTP divisions to establish guidelines for integrated surveillance.

2. Toward Integrated Training

    - NCHHSTP Office of the Director and divisions to provide training on PCSI for all center project officers and program consultants.

3. Toward Integrated Funding

    - CDC/NCHHSTP to fund pilot/demonstration projects of new PCSI opportunities.

    - CDC/NCHHSTP to fund evaluation and operational research on PCSI.

    - NCHHSTP divisions to collaborate on program announcements and post-award management.

    - NCHHSTP and partners to conduct national assessment of level of existing PCSI.

APPENDIX 2

Framework for Integrated Diagnostics

Diagnostic and laboratory issues that arise as a consequence of integrated provision of care are often complex and require careful planning. The schematic identifies points around the diagnostic pathway where decision points might occur to improve laboratory efficiency and service. Refer to the main text for a more detailed description of aspects for consideration at each step of the pathway.

PCSI Logic Model

Inputs
- Leadership
- Governance
- Policy and guidance
- Financial and human resources
- Collaboration with national partner organizations

NCHHSTP PCSI Activities
- Funding and Program Announcements
- Establish FOA standard of practice to ensure adoption of integrated language
- Incorporate PCSI language in FOAs to allow greater flexibility in use of funds
- Inventory FOA opportunities

Program Guidelines / Recommendations
- Issue / rollout integrated partner services guidelines
- Publish recommendations for integrated services to substance users

Surveillance
- Develop / publish integrated surveillance report
- Establish NCHHSTP confidentiality standards for data-sharing

CDC-Sponsored Training Courses
- Review existing curricula for integration opportunities
- Deliver integrated training at CDC and local level

NCHHSTP Work-Structure
- Establish PCSI meetings at the Division, Program Branch, and project officer level
- Support the MSM, IDU, surveillance, and corrections workgroups

Communication
- Publish White Paper
- Conduct PCSI sessions at national conferences
- Develop interactive web resources for NCHHSTP and partners

National Organization Activities
- Communication
- Training
- Partnerships
- Policy
- Evaluation

Shorter-Term Jurisdiction-level Outcomes*
- Flexibility to use funds for PCSI within jurisdiction
- Adoption of integrated partner services guidelines within jurisdiction
- Sharing and use of data across disease areas within jurisdiction
- PCSI-related knowledge and skills acquired through NCHHSTP-sponsored training programs
- Coordinated communication between grantees and POs across disease areas within jurisdiction
- Understanding of and support for PCSI among grantees

Shorter-Term NCHHSTP Outcomes
- Routine integration of PCSI language in FOAs
- Project officers collaborate across divisions to monitor overlapping grantee activities
- Divisions share and use data across disease areas
- Divisions communicate and collaborate on PCSI

Longer-Term Jurisdiction-level Outcomes
- Program collaboration across disease areas within jurisdiction
- Service integration across disease areas at point of service delivery

Longer-Term NCHHSTP Outcomes
- Institutionalization of PCSI in the day-to-day operations of NCHHSTP

Client-Level Public Health Impact
- Improved behavioral and health outcomes for clients
- Accessible, holistic, high-quality client services
- Greater opportunities to manage multiple epidemics

*Many of these shorter-term outcomes are derived from a list of PCSI barriers, Table 5, Green Paper[20] http://www.cdc.gov/nchhstp/programintegration/attachments/I-NCHHSTP-PCSIGreenPaper_508.pdf. Shorter-term outcomes are not assumed to occur simultaneously or at a fixed point in time, nor are they expected to occur to the same degree among all jurisdictions.

APPENDIX 4

Key Recommendations for PCSI Research

1. Evaluation of the Effectiveness of Integration

- NCHHSTP will conduct a survey to identify integration efforts already under-taken, best PCSI practices, and lessons learned in 2008–2009. Once it establishes such a baseline of integration, NCHHSTP will determine whether designing and carrying out a "proof of concept" trial using comparison communities is war-ranted.

2. Operational Research on Integration

- In accordance with Board of Scientific Counselors (BSC) recommendations, NCHHSTP laboratories will have a primary role in evaluating point-of-service screening tests before the tests receive FDA approval. NCHHSTP laboratories will develop models to determine test characteristics of public health value in the United States based on test sensitivity and specificity, the prevalence of the dis-ease a test screens for, and cost. CDC should promote the incorporation of test characteristics found to be of value and the widespread use of screening tests that incorporate these characteristics.

- CDC will help define the mix of screening services offered in the United States by determining the prevalence of coinfection in target populations and defining thresholds for when integration may be effective. Appropriate modeling will be used to develop thresholds before guidance is developed. NCHHSTP will undertake comorbidity studies so that subsequent recommendations are supported by data.

3. Research on Integrated Health Communication

- The BSC recommended, and NCHHSTP concurs, that a coordinated approach to health communication is appropriate. This approach should involve, at a mini-mum, all NCHHSTP divisions, NCHHSTP's Health Disparities Working Group, and NCHHSTP's Office of Communication. The group will choose target populations for integrated messages to develop a communication plan. They will also work to establish message priorities for targeted groups, design and evaluate integrated health- and service-based messages for specified populations, and evaluate the effectiveness of these messages in select communities according to specified outcome measures.